Save Your Life!
With the Power of pH Balance
by
Blythe Ayne, Ph.D.

Books by Blythe Ayne, Ph.D.

Nonfiction:
Love Is The Answer
45 Ways To Excellent Life
Horn of Plenty—The Cornucopia of Your Life
Life Flows on the River of Love
How to Save Your Life Series:
Save Your Life With The Power Of pH Balance
Save Your Life With The Phenomenal Lemon
Save Your Life with Stupendous Spices

Fiction:
The Darling Undesirables Series:
The Heart of Leo - short story prequel
The Darling Undesirables
Moons Rising
The Inventor's Clone
Heart's Quest

Short Story Collections:
5 Minute Stories
Lovely Frights for Lonely Nights

Children's Illustrated Books:
The Rat Who Didn't Like Rats
The Rat Who Didn't Like Christmas

Poetry:
Home & the Surrounding Territory

CD:
The Power of pH Balance –
Dr. Blythe Ayne Interviews Steven Acuff

Save Your Life!
With the Power of pH Balance

by

Blythe Ayne, Ph.D.

Save Your Life with the Power of pH Balance
Blythe Ayne, Ph.D.

Emerson & Tilman, Publishers
129 Pendleton Way #55
Washougal, WA 98671

Book & cover design by Blythe Ayne
All Text & Graphics © 2017 Blythe Ayne

Save Your Life with the Power of pH Balance

Other books in the save your life series:

Save Your Life With The Phenomenal Lemon

Save Your Life With Stupendous Spices

www.BlytheAyne.com

ISBN: 978-0-9827835-8-0

[1. HEALTH & FITNESS/Diet & Nutrition/Nutrition
2. HEALTH & FITNESS/Healing
3. HEALTH & FITNESS/Diseases/General

BIC: FM

First Edition

Your Free Gift

I want you to be healthy and happy. My gift to you, *Save Your Life with Stupendous Spices* helps you attain—and keep!—that goal.

Go to:
http://eepurl.com/bhNidj
to download
Save Your Life with Stupendous Spices

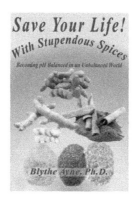

Save Your Life!
With the Power of pH Balance

Table of Contents:

Save Your Life!
With the Power of pH Balance

by Blythe Ayne, Ph.D.

Introduction

Why do gorgeous, fresh, clean little babies smell sweet? Because, chemically, they are predominately composed of sweet smelling, alkaline, mineralized water, and their bodies are pH balanced. To be in optimum, youthful health, we need to aspire to keep our bodies in pH balance too. pH Balance is critical to physical and mental health and well-being.

Chapter One

Food & pH Balance

"The countless names of illnesses do not really matter. What does matter is that they all come from the same root cause... too much tissue acid waste in the body!"
Theodore A. Baroody, N.D., D.C., Ph.D.

What causes acidic imbalance in your body? Stress, anxiety, worry, dietary habits and the environment—all contribute to your pH balance—or imbalance.

The pH scale is logarithmic, which means that pH 7 is ten times more alkaline than pH 6. pH 8 is 100 times more alkaline than pH 6, and pH 9 is 1,000 times more

Many health care practitioners and scientists around the world are in agreement that aging and disease are the direct result of the accumulation of acid waste products in the body. This belief is supported by scientific documentation.

Meats, sugar, white flour products, fried foods, soft drinks, processed foods, alcohol, dairy products, smoking, and drugs—all cause the body to become more acidic. Stress, whether mental or physical can also lead to acid deposits in the body.

Our highly acidic dietary intake is fueling the plethora of diseases and emotional melt down we see on earth today.

We begin the twenty-first century with hope and fear, knowing we must figure out how to take action or suffer the consequences of not getting the full advantage in this amazing and wonderful life. Laying claim to a mindfully consumed diet is one of the most important steps toward this goal.

Why isn't food just as nutritious and life sustaining as it ever was? The short answer is because we have roared ahead with actions and behaviors that have had serious consequences. We have polluted our waters and air, and contaminated our soil, without understanding the results and outcome of our actions.

In this first chapter on food, we'll explore several avenues of concern, and then look at an action plan that will make you feel empowered, and, when put into action will make you healthier. It's a win-win action plan, because just as you are caring and thoughtful of your body and your body's health, these same conscientious behaviors benefit the entire planet.

alkaline than pH 6. For a little perspective, cola is pH 2.5, meaning it is over 10,000 times more acid than most tap water, and 100,000 times more acid than your blood at pH 7.365.

WHAT IS A HEALTHY, BALANCED pH?

Your body is constantly working, 24-7 to maintain a delicate balance between acidity and alkalinity. Everything you take in moves toward one end or the other of the pH teeter-totter. And not only everything you ingest, but also the very air you breath and the emotions you experience—all contribute to your pH (which stands for "potential Hydrogen").

Considering the teeter-totter analogy, we can say that the kid at the acidic end is a bit chubby and the kid at the alkaline end is thin ...

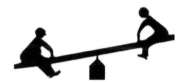

0 to 6.9 = Acidic   7 = neutral pH   7.1 to 14 = Alkaline

So to balance the teeter-totter, the acidic kid needs to scooch in a bit and the alkaline kid needs to scooch out.

The pH scale runs from 0 to 14. Our blood must maintain a slightly alkaline 7.365 pH, OR WE CEASE TO BE. You will have a fun ride through life when keeping your pH neutral. Seven days a week, 365 day of the year, our blood pH needs to be 7.365!

Although that probably doesn't sound too complicated or difficult, nothing worth having is without its challenges. In simplest terms, this means eat mindfully!

For instance, if we average the components of a typical fast food sandwich, it will come out at between

2 to maybe 3 highly acid-forming. And unless you have a side order of a head of lettuce, you are then trying to get through your day highly acidic.

This is really weighing down the chubby kid's end of the teeter-totter. Drinking coffee? Highly acid-forming with a rating of 1.5. Adding cream or sugar? Take another .5 off of the 1.5 for each, which equals .5. Or a soda? Acid-forming at about 2 to 2.5. Diet soda (never mind the cancer producing aspect of the non-food of artificial sweeteners - a whole other topic!) is very highly acid-forming at a rating of 1!

You never, ever again need to wonder why you have acid indigestion.

EAT YOUR VEGETABLES!

Dr. Baroody, author of *Alkalize or Die*, one of the foremost proponents of pH balance, recommends an 80-20 alkaline-forming diet. That is to say, have 80% of your nutritional intake at not below 5.0 pH. Almost all vegetables range from 5-7 pH, and are alkaline-forming and almost all fruits range from 6-7.5 pH, also alkaline-forming.

Each number on the pH scale is logarithmic. Something that is a 2 acid-forming is ten times more so than something that is a 3, and one-hundred times more acid-forming than a 4.

The 80-20 game plan will help arm your hard-working body against the acidic environmental and emotional influences taxing your system that is predominate in our world today.

WHAT FOODS ARE ACID-FORMING?

In simplest terms, most high protein foods and carbohydrates are acid-forming. Fruits and vegetables are alkaline-forming.

Interestingly ... although animal products (meat, fish, poultry, dairy) are predominately alkaline, they are acid-forming in the human body when consumed.

Conversely, although a lemon is obviously acidic, it is just about the best source of alkaline-forming ash in the human body you can get!

At the end of the book, you will find an Alkaline Acid Chart. You may have seen similar charts which run acid to alkaline (because acid is the lower number on the pH scale). But as the focus of this book is to become more aware of alkaline and alkalizing food and beverages, I've listed these first on the chart, so you can readily see them).

FOOD COMBINING

Although we want to eat what we want to eat when we want to eat it, there are a few fundamentals about certain combinations of food that show care and thoughtfulness of the chemistry and biology of your body. If you begin to take these into consideration the benefits over time will reinforce your conscious shift in habits!

The combinations of foods you eat now are simply an accumulation of habits. And, even though it may seem like something resembling work to change your habits, a little challenge makes you feel great once the challenge is mastered.

Do not feel overwhelmed or discouraged by this information. Rather, take one or two suggestions that resonate with you and begin to incorporate them into your daily diet habits. How much better you will feel over time is the pay-off for changing poor habits.

I have a friend who is an energetic, funny, charming man. A while back, though, I noticed a change in his usually quick-witted, on-the-go behavior. He was moving slower and seemed depressed. When he failed to make a single pun in a conversation, I knew something was amiss.

I asked him what was up, and he told me he'd been diagnosed with gout and not only was he physically in pain, but, he said, the diagnosis really knocked him for a loop emotionally because he felt that gout was "an old man's disease."

I told him not to be sad, but to be happy because he had power over the situation. I then suggested that he not only to cut down (or even better, cut out) eating red meat, which any doctor would tell him (and his did) but not to eat meat and potatoes together.

He said he was willing to try anything—which, he admitted, it wasn't that long ago that he could not have imagined he'd ever hear himself say such a thing.

Long story short, he really did shift these two habits and within a month was feeling so much better that his punning redoubled—which was the only down side of his improved health.

So, without further preamble, here are some basics about combinations of food:

Melons are extremely alkaline-forming and are very good for you. They need to be eaten alone or at least 20 minutes before any other food. As they digest quickly, if they are held up by other foods they quickly decompose and ferment.

Don't eat fruits and vegetables at the same time. Fresh fruits digest rapidly, at the most, in a little over an hour, and some vegetable can take as long as 3 hours to digest.

Avoid combining starches with fruits. Fruits like bananas, dates or prunes with a starch such as bread will ferment in the stomach, and is moderately acid-forming.

But do eat starchy foods with vegetables, like rice with steamed vegetables or bread with fresh salad. This combination is moderately alkaline-forming.

Do not have two starches in the same meal (bread and potatoes, rice and potatoes).

Starches do not combine with proteins, as proteins are extremely acid-forming. When protein starts digesting, hydrochloric acid is secreted in the stomach, while, at the same time, starch neutralizes hydrochloric acid. The extremely acid-forming process of putrefaction is the result, and toxins and illness manifest in this climate. Examples of what to avoid are the common practice of meat and potatoes, beans and bread.

Do not have more than one high-protein at a meal.

Light proteins, such as cottage cheese, yogurt, nuts, and tofu combine well with fruit or non-starchy vegetables.

Beans with grains form a complete, healthy protein. Black beans and rice, yum!

The enzymes pepsin and rennin in milk coagulate milk in the stomach. Other foods you eat with milk are then prevented from digestion. The coagulated milk clings to other foods and insulates them from digestion and it all begins to putrefy. This is acid-forming.

> *"As houses stored with provision are*
> *full of mice, so the bodies of those*
> *who eat much are full of disease."*
> **Diogenes**

ADDICTIONS

Sugar/Caffeine

It is easier to get a sugar loaded, caffeine based beverage in our world than it is to get a drink of pure water. We drink caffeine loaded coffee, tea and soda, and mistake the adrenaline charge as energizing and relief from thirst.

Our biggest selling and most consumed soft drink is 10,000 times more acid than our blood, with a pH of 2.5. Alkaline, stored in your body that needs to be used elsewhere is sacrificed to the urgent call of the adrenaline that floods your system, every time you take a sip. The 'high' is not entirely dissimilar to the high any drug user experiences, which is a dangerous and artificial sensory elevation.

Thirty-two glasses of neutral pH water are needed to balance one glass of a cola beverage, the active ingredient being Phosphoric Acid.

Eating Disorders

Why is there burgeoning obesity in the world? The food we eat, its quantity and quality, has, of course, a "large" affect on weight. But also, as the over-acid body has made a habit of pirating calcium from the bones and teeth to neutralize the excess toxic acid waste, there is another reason we accrue fat.

When your body is faced with a shortage of options of what to do with the excess acid when it materializes faster than your body can flush it out, your body dumps toxic wastes into fatty deposits, as far away from the organs and heart as possible—hips, back, chest, thighs, upper arms, belly.

Dr. Robert O. Young, author of *The pH Miracle*, has noted that the body has to protect itself from the excess sugar we consume, and so it co-opts fat to encase it and protect us from it.

Take a look at a very few world obesity statistics to get a notion of the "plague of obesity" earth's human population is in the midst of.

Percent of Obese Population:

Kuwait	42.8%
Belize	34.9%
Jordan	34.3%
South Africa	33.5%
U.S.	33%
Mexico	32.8%
UK	26.9%
Australia	26.8%
Spain	26.6%
Russia	26.5%
Canada	26.2%

(Statistics from www.NationMaster.com. Go to this site to see the shocking statistics of obesity all around the world.)

So obesity, and weight gain in general, is not because of calories, *per se.* An approach of reducing calories will not work to bring about a lifelong healthy weight. Healthy weight is about an alkaline-forming diet. Obesity arises from an acidic diet. The relationship between weight and calories is more accurately the relationship between weight and acidity. In general terms, acidic foods have more calories in them.

But, to repeat, it is not:

excess calories = excess weight

it *is:*

excess acid = excess weight

With the exception of folks who have a high metabolism, (who may still be very acidic and unhealthy) the rest of us struggle almost helplessly with our weight—unless and until we learn to balance our pH.

Your body works valiantly to keep the excess of acid, or acidic environment, away from your vital organs. (Losing this battle is why there are so many heart attacks and strokes). What your body must do is find a place to stick that acid, and so it goes into your fat cells, as fat is a pretty good medium to keep acid away from the organs.

When fat cells fill, a person gets fatter, and looks bloated. Even thin people with acidic imbalance often get "puffy" looking.

The effectiveness with which your nervous system can operate is subject to a correct pH. By eating and living in a way that causes imbalances to your internal pH balance literally "kills the messenger."

WHAT CAN I DO?

- A simple test to see if you're too acidic is to pinch the skin on your back. It does not matter if you're a skinny-minnie or over-weight. If you are acidic, you'll discover that you almost cannot get a purchase on the skin on your back.

I've had very thin people say "that's because I'm too skinny" and overweight people say, "that's because I'm too fat." But no, it's because of being too acidic and, again, the body is doing everything in its power to move the acid away from internal organs and out to the fat layer under the skin, filling the fat cells with the poisonous acid.

SOME DIETARY CONSIDERATIONS:

- Eat only if you are actually hungry.
- Keep meals simple.
- Eat foods at room temperature.
- Eat juicy foods prior to concentrated foods.
- Eat raw foods before cooked foods.

- Eat more raw foods in the summer.
- Avoid refined foods and sweeteners (The so-call "White Foods" white bread, white rice, white sugar, etc.).
- Chew, chew, chew ... then chew some more. Allow the alkaline-forming enzyme, ptyalin to begin digestion in the mouth, which is as nature intends. *The more you chew, the more alkaline your nutrition becomes.*
- Avoid drinking while eating. Beverages, even water, interfere with the process of ptyalin.
- Drink, in ounces, half your weight in water. If you weigh 150 pounds, drink 75 ounces (9.5 glasses) of water per day. Drink an additional glass of water for every 10 pounds you desire to drop. I'm sure you can do the math in you own case.
- As a General Rule: The longer the list of contents on the container label, the less you want that concoction inside you.
- Do not eat when tired, anxious, angry, overheated, chilled, in pain, upset or with a fever.
- Acquire a good set of stainless steel pots and pans.
- Cook on medium to low heat to conserve nutrients.
- Grow and eat sprouts.
- Become an expert at the most important exercise of all - push yourself away from the table a little bit

hungry. It takes 20 minutes for your brain to get the message from your stomach "I'M FULL!"

• Soak your fruits and veggies in a solution of sea salt and water for ten minutes. This will draw out pesticides, kill bug eggs, and neutralize acid contaminates. You can get sea salt anywhere; from your bulk food rows at you warehouse grocery store, to your local Whole Foods health food store. Or, at least use table salt (although sea salt is profoundly preferred as it has a full compliment of natural and much needed alkaline minerals in its content).

• Dr. Baroody suggests soaking fruits and veggies in a sink full of water with a tablespoon of bleach in the water.

• Feel hungry? First of all, drink down one, and better yet, two glasses of water. Many of your "hunger signals" are actually thirst signals. We do not drink enough water, and because of this, we do not have an educated awareness of the difference between a hunger signal and a "dying of thirst" signal.

• Consider taking alkalizing supplements, enzyme supplements, organic calcium and magnesium, colloidal minerals, and vitamins A and D.

• Supplement with alkaline substances such as vegetable juices, virtually any greens, liquid chlorophyll, powdered or fresh barley, wheat grasses, spirulina, chlorella, calcium and magnesium supplements, alkaline water.

• Get acid-alkaline test strips—available at health food stores and perhaps your local pharmacy. Although there's debate around whether one can get relevant information from urine pH testing, I believe you can become more familiar with your own chemistry and that the pH test strips help inform you of your body's pH.

• Testing at the same time each morning, for instance, familiarizes you with the effect of diet and stressors and regular testing is another tool in your tool box on the path to radiant health. It is interesting to see the literal effects of your body throwing off acidic wastes and then becoming more balanced as it moves from over acidic to more alkaline.

• Choose a diet in favor of alkaline-forming foods to live a long and healthy life!

• Add An alkaline-forming Super Food:

• There are some foods that are such complete nutrition, and alkalizing to boot, that it is highly recommended you look into adding them to your diet. Be sure to do additional research around super foods, and/or consult with your health food store pharmacist, your homeopath, or naturopath, as, for instance, some people are allergic to bee products.

- Bee Pollen - a complete, highly alkaline food. You could live on bee pollen alone.
- Royal Jelly - highly alkaline.
- Chlorophyll products - the only difference between chlorophyll and blood is the center of the molecule. Chlorophyll builds your blood and alkalizes your system. There are many forms and brands. Consult your health food store.
- Sea Vegetables (aka: seaweed) - grow in both marine salt waters as well as fresh water lakes and seas on coral reefs or on rocks. They will grow at great depths as long as sunlight penetrates to where they are, as they require sunlight.
- Sea vegetables have the broadest range of minerals of any food, containing the same minerals that are found in human blood. They are an excellent source of iodine, vitamin K, the B-vitamin folate, and magnesium, and a good source of iron, calcium, and the B-vitamins riboflavin and pantothenic acid. Sea vegetables also contain lignans, plant compounds that have cancer-protective properties.

Chapter Two

Water & pH Balance

*"One of the main causes of fatigue,
toxemia, constipation, and premature
aging is simply that most people
don't drink enough water."*
Sue Pollock, ND

Water is the elixir of life. The more we understand the various amazing properties of water, and employ what we learn, *A minimum amount of water per day is one ounce per pound of body weight. If you are ill, detoxifying, or intentionally losing*

the better the quality of our lives, and the life of the planet.

Water is involved with every metabolic process, electrical exchange, biochemical pathway, and physical and mental action in the body. It extracts nutrients from food, transports these nutrients to the blood, replenishes vital fluids, and helps detoxify your body.

Three quarters of your body is water. Your muscles are 70% water, your blood 82% to 90% water, your bones contain up to 35% water, your liver is 90% water, and your brain 85% water!

If your body doesn't get enough water, it must recycle what it already has by re-filtering it through the kidneys, which places an undue burden on the kidneys and the liver.

Dehydration is one of the main causes of fluid retention and is often the cause of chronic pains such as headaches, arthritis, and a host of others. This is because of the concentration of acids and toxins recirculating the body, and also because of the drying of the lubricating layer of interfacial tissue, causing friction, which exacerbates tissue inflammation and pain.

In direct proportion to the amount of water that enters the stomach, the hormone/neurotransmitter "motilin" is secreted by the intestinal tract, which can be measured in circulating blood.

Motilin produces rhythmic contractions of the intestines known as peristalsis. But as motilin is only secreted in an amount in direct proportion to the volume of water that enters the stomach, dehydration results and may often be the cause of abdominal pain, constipation, and colitis.

The osmotic flow of water through cell membrane generates hydroelectric energy, which is converted and stored in energy pools. This energy is important for all cellular processes, including neurotransmission.

Japan has been at the forefront of developing and researching restructured water. Devices called water ionizers split alkaline minerals and acid minerals in regular

weight, consider doubling that amount.

Also consider a water treatment system which alkalizes your water. Alkaline water charged with negative ions is an antioxidant, scavenging free radicals and neutralizing acids and toxic substances, which are positively charged, in the blood and tissues.

A water ionizer attached to your tap or to your cold water line takes in regular tap water which has both acid and alkaline minerals in it. The system then produces water with a pH value of 9 or higher, while at the same time separately producing acidic tap water by electrical means. Japanese scientists at Shiga University suggest that optimum water needs to be at pH 8.5 or above.

Published Japanese research provides case histories and statistics of alkalized water successfully treating cancers, arthritis, immune dysfunction, hangovers, aging, tissue detoxification, among many other health concerns.

Here are some brief excerpts from extensive reports and scientific studies data:

"During my long years of servicing pre-eclamptic toxemia cases, I found that the women with pre-eclamptic toxemia who consumed antioxidant water deliver healthier babies with stronger muscles. A survey report carried out on babies in this group showed intelligence above average."

Prof. Watanabe Ifao, Watanabe Hospital

"The wonder of antioxidant water is its ability to neutralize toxins, but it is not a medicine. The difference is that medicine can only apply to each individual case, whereas antioxidant water can be consumed generally. I introduce a heart disease case and how he was cured.

"The patient was a 35 years old male suffering from vascular heart disease. For five years, his health deteriorated. During those five years, he had been in and out of the hospital five or six times. He had undergone high-tech examinations, including angiogram by injecting VINYL via the vein into the heart.

"He consulted and sought treatment from many good doctors where later he underwent a major surgical operation. However, he relapsed, and the attack appeared to be more severe.

"At that time, a relative of the patient came across an antioxidant water processor. The patient's illness responded well and he is now on the road to recovery."

Prof. Kuwata Keijiroo,
Doctor of Medicine

"This patient suffered 10 years of eczema and could not be cured, even under specialist treatment. After the war, this

water with a pH value of 5 or lower, (which is an excellent plant water and household disinfectant). It filters your water of impurities, including chlorine. Its magnetic process produces water molecules which allow for superior hydration. The latest alkaline water ionizers employ Far Infra red (FIR) emitting ceramics to help energize and disinfect the water.

Water can also be alkalized by adding alkaline minerals/water alkalizing drops, although effective for alkalizing your water, they do not clear or ionize the water.

patient's lower limbs suffered acute eczema, which later became chronic. He was repeatedly treated in a skin specialist hospital.

"He suffered severe itchiness, which, when scratched led to bleeding. During the last 10 years, he was seen and treated by many doctors. When I first examined him, his lower limb around the joints was covered with vesicles. Weeping occurred owing to serum exuding from the vesicles.

"I advised him to try consuming antioxidant water. He bought a unit and consumed the antioxidant water religiously and used the acidic water to bathe the affected areas. After 2 weeks of treatment the vesicles dried up. The eczema was completely cleared without any relapse after one-and-one-half months."

Prof. Tamura Tatsuji, Keifuku Rehabilitation Center
The alkaline water neutralizes acidic elements, which the body then eliminates. People all over the world using alkalized water have reported better digestion, weight loss, increase in energy, migraine headache reduction, disappearance of eczema, improvement in chronic fatigue, arthritis, M.S., depression, etc., etc., etc. In clinical studies, live

blood analysis which showed acid crystals and clumping of cells before drinking alkalized water showed that the acid crystals had disappeared after drinking the water for a mere two weeks.

Water is more than simply a thirst quencher and nutrient transport system. It also functions as digestion aid, solvent, dilutor, dilator, waste disposal system, electrical and chemical conduit, energy combustor, lubricant, coolant and latent heat bank. There is even research around the idea that water is the repository of emotion. Drinking the best quality, pH healthy water appears to be, in numerous ways, the better part of wisdom.

In a University of Washington study, drinking one glass of water when feeling hungry stopped the hunger pangs in 98% of the dieters surveyed.

The main cause of daytime fatigue is a lack of water.

Research shows that about 8-10 glasses of water a day may significantly ease back pain and joint pain for up to 80% of sufferers.

If the average person drank a mere 5 glasses of plain water a day, the risk of getting breast cancer is decreased by as much as 79%, colon cancer by 45% and bladder cancer by 50%. (Water in your coffee, tea,

*"We have observed various kinds of
water crystals in our laboratory and
have found that water containing
minerals in a healthy balance tends to
turn out well-ordered hexagonal
crystals.*

*"Energetically speaking, we believe
that water needs to have good Hado to
create a beautiful crystal. "*

Dr. Masaru Emoto, Messages From Water

POISON IN YOUR WATER

Chlorine is added to municipal water supplies. This is a disinfectant that hardens arteries,
destroys proteins, irritates skin and sinus conditions, or aggravates asthma, allergies, and respiratory
problems.

Chloroform is a by-product of chlorination. It
causes excessive free radical formation, which causes
aging. Normal cells mutate, and cholesterol oxidizes.
It is a known cancer-producing carcinogen.

Dichloro acetic acid (DCA) is a chlorine by-product. It alters cholesterol metabolism and has caused
liver cancer in lab animals.

Another by-product of chlorination is MX, found in all chlorinated water, which is known to cause genetic mutations according to the Environmental Protection Agency (EPA).

Aluminum is sometimes used as a clarifying agent in water. Excesses of aluminum are medically linked with a number of diseases and disorders, including Alzheimer's.

Research has shown that chlorinated water is the direct cause of 9% of all bladder cancers and 15% of all rectal cancers in the US.

Through your skin, your largest organ, you absorb more chlorine in a 10-minute shower than by drinking 8 glasses of the same water! A warm shower opens up your pores, and causes your skin to

(except some herbal teas) sodas, etc., does not count towards daily water needs as they are so acidic they contribute to the problem, not the solution). (stats: Stress Management Institute)

Only a 2% drop *in the amount of water in your body can bring on mental confusion, short-term memory loss, being unable to focus, and forgetting how to do simple sequential activities.*

act like a sponge. As a result, you not only inhale chlorine vapors, you also absorb them through your skin, directly into your bloodstream absorbing up to six times more chlorine than drinking the water.

Chlorinated shower water irritates eyes, sinuses, throat, skin, and lungs. Long term effects are the aging process of free radical formation, hardened arteries, difficulty metabolizing cholesterol, increased potential for cancers, and increasing the odds of manifesting genetic mutations in your as yet unborn children, among others.

There is also evidence that chlorine destroys protein in your body. If you suffer from sinus conditions, allergies, skin rashes or emphysema, chlorinated water makes your condition worse.

IMPORTANT CAUTIONS REGARDING PURIFIED AND DISTILLED WATER

Water is boiled, evaporated and the vapor condensed to produce distilled water. Cooking foods in distilled water pulls the minerals out of them and lowers their nutrient value. Many metals are dissolved by distilled water.

Purified water, or reverse osmosis, is free of dissolved minerals. Because of this it actively absorbs toxic substances from the body and eliminates them. Drinking purified water is beneficial for a few weeks when you are detoxing your system, but fasting using purified water can be dangerous because of the rapid loss of electrolytes (sodium, potassium, chloride) and trace minerals, deficiencies which can cause heart beat irregularities and high blood pressure.

According to the U.S. Environmental Protection Agency (EPA), "purified" water, being essentially mineral-free, is very aggressive as it dissolves substances with which it comes in contact. Notably, carbon dioxide from the air is rapidly absorbed, making the water acidic and even more aggressive.

Soft drinks are made from purified water and are toxic. Studies have shown that heavy consumers of soft drinks (with or without sugar) spill huge amounts of calcium, magnesium and other trace minerals into their urine. This mineral loss leads to osteoporosis, osteoarthritis, hypothyroidism, coronary artery disease, high blood pressure, and a long list of diseases generally associated with premature aging.

There is a correlation between the consumption of purified water and the incidence of cardiovascular disease. Cells, tissues and organs will do anything to avoid being in this acid environment, including removing minerals from the skeleton.

Drinking purified water exclusively you will eventually develop multiple mineral deficiencies if no bio-available mineral supplements are taken.

IONIZED WATER—
POTENTIAL HEALTH BENEFITS

ORP stands for "Oxygen Reduction Potential." Potential energy is energy that is stored and ready to be put to work. "Potential" in the term ORP refers to the electrical potential expressed in voltage. This energy is measured in millivolts with an ORP meter that reads the very slight voltage in water, actually measuring the presence of oxidizing and reducing agents, the Oxidation Reduction "Potential."

High pH water has more reducing agents (-ORP) and low pH water has more oxidizing agents (+ORP). Normal tap water in the U.S. measures +200 to +600mv. Ionized water measures ORP -250mv or lower (the lower the ORP number = the more negative ions = the more alkaline = the better). This produces the antioxidant effect in water through the creation of the negative hydroxyl ion, which can then more readily penetrate to the cellular level and remove acid toxins. When water becomes stagnant by staying in dams, pipes and bottles, the ORP becomes very positive. When water bounces over rocks or a waterfall the ORP becomes negative.

Ionized water producing hydroxyl ions helps with oxygen production, neutralizing harmful free radicals, increasing your energy level, correcting your body's acid/alkaline balance, hydrating cells, and potentially reducing many of the symptoms of aging. Millions of dollars are spent on the antioxidant vitamins A, C and E which, if the body is too acidic, may not be bio-accessible, and millions more are spent on buying bottled water that is over one-hundred times more acidic than regular water, and which is unable to be ionized because all of the essential alkalizing minerals have been taken out.

What vitamins A, C and E have in common with ionized water are they are capable of carrying oxygen with an extra electron attached. These hydroxyl ions in the ionized water seek out and neutralize free radicals, which cause damage to our cells and bring about disease and premature aging. When the hydroxyl ions have neutralized the free radicals, the result is your body is rich in oxygen and energy.

Oxygen helps destroy cancer cells, removes waste, carries nutrients and aids in resisting bacteria and viruses that invade your body, but in our modern world oxygen levels are depleted due to stress, environmental pollution, diet and lack of exercise.

A high positive ORP (such as found in most bottled and city water) creates oxidation and accelerates the aging process. In comparison, when you drink clean, ionized water you are drinking a powerful and natural antioxidant that renews you at the cellular level. If you make fresh organic juice you will have an antioxidant with a -250 ORP. Yet ionized water will give this ORP or even lower. If you still drink coffee etc., then make it with ionized water, and cook with ionized water, as it hydrates, and neutralizes acids, it enhances the flavor, while being much healthier.

Feeling over-tired, weak, restless, frustrated, stiff, overwhelmed, unfocused or confused are often early warning signs that your body is no longer able to cope with its toxic overload. Your body tries to reduce the effect of this excess acid by taking calcium from the bones, and magnesium needed for heart health. Ionized water helps your body balance its pH.

If your body's communication channels break down, cancerous cells may appear, organs will shrink and degenerate. Because it is very alkaline, ionized water dissolves accumulated acid waste and helps to restore balance.

Reducing over-acidity is your first line of defense in fighting any disease. Throughout the ages we have known to drink water that has been moving in streams and rivers, bouncing over rocks, and which is free from chemicals. In Grecian times water was stored over night in copper and brass urns to cause ionization, the water became clear and sweet due to the electrolytic reaction that took place overnight.

> *"When you drink alkaline water, you are drinking water with excess oxygen, not in the form of O2, but in the form of OH - which is very stable because it is mated with positively ionized alkaline minerals. Two of these hydroxyl ions can form a water molecule (H2O) and give out one oxygen atom. The alkaline mineral is used to detoxify poisonous acid compounds and when that happens the hydroxyl ion is freed to supply excess oxygen to the cells to prevent the development of cancer."*
> **Sang Whang, Reverse Aging**

WHAT CAN I DO?

• Acid indigestion? Before grabbing the pill *du jour,* drink down a glass of water. Keep in mind that water is more alkaline than the acid you're battling and it has the potential to neutralize the acid. The more alkaline your water, the more powerful the remedy. Notice how most if not all of your acidic sensation fades away after drinking a glass of water.

• In an effort to solve the problem of worsening public water quality, more and more people are turning to water in plastic containers. However, water in plastic bottles is highly acidic, missing the essential alkalizing minerals.

• Get alkalizing drops and bottle your own water, using stainless steel or glass bottles. *NOT* plastic! Or invest in one of the many options of filtered water bottles.

• Install a de-chlorinating shower filter and a kitchen sink filter, and purchase a de-chlorinating bath ball. This is especially important for children, whose little bodies absorb the negative effects of chlorine even more than adults.

• Install a water treatment system that alkalizes your water. Alkaline water is well worth the investment in health and longevity!

• Use alkaline soaps and laundry products.

Chapter Three

Air & pH Balance

Our planet's air, water and soil are all profoundly contaminated, that is to say, acidic, due to our short-sighted abuses. Every exhaust fume, every chimney plume, every field of cows producing carbon dioxide and CFCs is bringing our planet—and taking us with it - to it's knees.

Molecules in the Air
A plastic chair and plastic wall coverings accelerate mental fatigue.

Objects covered in polyethylene produce fields of between 5 and 10,000 volts/meter. A space enclosed by polyethylene can skyrocket the rate to 100,000 volts/meter.

Where once clear air and streams and rivers produced all the negative ions we needed, now they do not. Chemical factories from around the world contaminate Ocean air.

Gases, dust, chemical fumes enter the body as positive ions, trapping and constraining the tiny negative ions from accomplishing their energetic purpose, leaving us needing to replenish our negative ions, which is life energy itself.

An air ionizer creates ions that remove microscopic particles from the air by changing the chemical properties of particles. An ionizer creates negative ions (alkaline) via electricity, which flood the room and seek out positively charged particles, (acidic) such as dust, dander, bacteria, pollen, mold, smoke, chemical vapors, and many other allergens.

These positively charged particles, once bonded to the negative ion, are now too heavy to float around and become inhaled. The harmful airborne particles fall to the floor where they can be readily cleaned up.

Phenomenon such as lightning and waterfalls generate negative ions and ozone. This is the fresh, invigorating smell (and feeling!) you experience in an electrical storm or white rapids. Ozone is a naturally occurring gas related to oxygen. Insulation in our buildings interferes with atmospheric air circulation, dust and mold collects inside heating and air conditioning ducts, indoor humidity allows bacteria to thrive.

An air ionizer helps restore balance to your indoor environment. Ozone that is created when negative ions are generated deodorizes the air and breaks down pollution into harmless components, making it difficult for germs to grow.

With the ionization of air, your body receives ionized nitrogen and oxygen that is immediately available to facilitate your energy conversion and storage. Ionized nitrogen acts on your cellular communication system, dilating

Some synthetics in clothing can set up a field that repels negative ions away from you.

Think about what a baseball cap does -it interferes with the flow of electrical synapse right where (one would think ... if one can) you want it most.

Dry cleaning fluid, Carbon Tetrachloride, enters the body through the pores and can cause chemical sensitivities. Be sure to air out dry cleaned clothes when you get them home to allow the chemical to dissipate.

Formaldehyde is present in may products, wood paneling, chip board flooring, carpet.

blood vessels to maintain a strong nutrient transport system.

John Hamaker, ecologist, pointed out in the 1980's that we are making an ice age with the massive acid wastes we dump into our environment. In an ice age, glaciers crush rocks to dust and remineralize, that is to say, alkalize, the soil so that trees and foliage can grow.

Our salvation is in reforestation and remineralization with crushing gravel to rock dust, which will not only potentially forestall an ice-age, but will produce alkaline organic produce and grains, bring lakes back to life, and reverse the climatic changes we are now witnessing.

EMF'S AND pH BALANCE

Electromagnetic Frequencies (EMFs) are an unseen bombardment to our delicate (while at the same time tough!) bio-electrical system. There is extensive research on the influences of all the electrical, magnetic consequences of the burgeoning plethora of televisions, radios, computers, cell phones, household, workplace and school electricity zooming and boomeranging through us, 24-7.

Never in all the time humanity has inhabited this planet have we had such influences on our bio-beings. The accumulative influence is acidic. More and ever more we need alkaline balance. There are a variety of products on the market which claim to be EMF neutralizing, which may sound rather woo-woo. But why not stick one on your cell phone or your kid's computer? If, by chance, it prevents just one cancer, or one school shooting, it would be entirely worth it.

Talcum (silicon dioxide) has been linked to serious physical problems, including cancer, etc.

Dioxin is a highly acid-forming poison in cigarettes and cigars (along with 2000 other chemicals in processed tobacco).

"There are 230 million times more radio frequencies in the air today than there were in 1939, which are increasing exponentially.
"The computer era is creating an unseen plague of acid-reaction

frequencies sailing through us, interacting negatively with the chemicals and heavy metal pollutants already in the air. These stressors form acid reactions in the body."

Dr. Theodore Baroody

WHAT CAN I DO?

- Yoga, and/or tai chi to center, calm, heal, oxygenate, and to fully engage your "gears" that is to say, life force, or "prana" in East Indian tradition and "chi" in Chinese

- Drive less, car pool

- Plant a tree, or contribute/donate to reforestation

Chapter Four

A Bit of Science

"It is not the germs we need worry about.
It is our inner terrain."
Louis Pasteur

It is very challenging to make a point about pH balance without getting into a bit of science, but I will do my best to make it "user friendly."

The pH scale runs from 0 to 14. A rating of "0" is fully acidic,

What is an ion?
An "ion" is any atom that has a positive or a negative charge. A positively charged ion will seek a negatively charged one to unite with and turn into usable energy.

and a rating of "14" fully alkaline. The magic elixir of our lives is blood, which must maintain a slightly alkaline pH or the host dies. As the body is completely dedicated to preventing this from happening, it does everything in its power to keep the blood at never more than 7.4. pH.

When your body breaks down (metabolizes) what you put into it, it yields an "ash" or waste material that is very informative about how your body was able to put to use the materials you gave it to build with.

The goal, if you love your body, is to have this ash inform you that the supplies provided were pH balancing.

Why? Because, as previously mentioned, your body is somewhere between 50% to 80% water. This water allows nutrients, oxygen and biochemicals to be transported about to every nook and cranny of your physical being.

If this medium is too acidic or too alkaline, the entire system will break down and not function. Our usual term for this process is "disease" with many, many entries, as we know, under that heading. However, they are virtually all the result of an over-acidic pH imbalance.

Diets high in protein, fat and carbohydrates and low in greens and raw food, stress the digestive system and inhibit proper digestion, and also overload the immune system with incompletely digested macromolecules and toxins, all negatively compounded by high intake of food additives, pesticides and stimulating foods.

Because the result of every move you make is positive, the molecules are left holding a positive charge, and need to unite with negative ions to produce more energy.

The bulk of the diet of industrialized, omnivorous countries consists of foods that leave an acidic ash when metabolized, and this imbalance will slowly but steadily corrode your body, just as an acid rain on a forest will slowly but surely cause it to die.

All of your regulatory systems—breathing, circulation, digestion, hormone production, perspiration, elimination—have the same core "job description"—to balance the pH. They all work every single moment of every single day and night to remove caustic acid residues from your body tissues, without damaging the living cells. But ... if your pH deviates from a balanced midpoint, your precious cells become poisoned by their own toxic waste, and they die.

Did you know that you have 60,000 miles of veins and arteries, into which an acidic pH eats like acid on marble? This acidic destruction can possibly take quiet years to manifest, but when it does, it is dramatic ... heart attacks, strokes, obesity ... so on and so on.

> "Most things that go between our lips these days are acidic, our lifestyles are acid-producing ... our body has to work hard to give us alkaline blood."
> **Sue Pollock, ND**

Your blood, which is the only transport system for nutrients to every part of your body, passes through the heart at a rate of 130 liters per hour. If your blood shifts slightly from its required pH, beneficial microforms die, and aggressive microforms, sustained by an acidic environment, begin to multiply and mutate, becoming parasitic, pathogenic agents.

The kidneys filter one liter of blood per minute. When clogged with acid wastes, it produces painful kidney stones and/or an inflamed bladder.

Your blood flies through your liver every three minutes, which is accomplishing an amazing job of filtering all those toxic wastes and acids from your bloodstream.

At the same time, it is producing enzymes to alkalize your blood. Liver Function Tests often show an elevation of these enzymes, confirming that the liver is working overtime in its effort to reduce acid wastes and toxins, and therefore it hasn't had time in which to do its many other functions.

Your poor little liver then, in a virtually frenzy of being overtaxed, throws excess acid wastes into joints as a "safe place" because there they cannot be introduced into your organs. So, instead of dying, you get arthritis, fibromyalgia, or a host of other joint and muscular problems.

"When we consider organic life in the light of biophysics, we find that electrical

*phenomena are at the root of all cellular
life and we conclude that (at the core) of
everything is an electrical charge."*
Dr. J. Belot, French Scientist

Your body also alkalizes your blood via the lungs through respiration. Have you noticed that when you're sick, you increase your breathing rate? This is to get more oxygen in to support the alkaline environment in the blood and tissues so you will get well.

Acidity is buffered in your body with alkaline minerals, the most abundant being calcium, which, as we know, resides in bones and teeth. Bone and tooth disorders are not as much caused by lack of calcium or dairy products as an excess of acid pH, so that the body must steal calcium from your bones and teeth to alkalize it.

Another important alkalizing mineral is magnesium, which stress uses up with impunity. Calcium and magnesium have a symbiotic relationship, supporting one another.

Low calcium and magnesium causes us to become stressed more easily, which causes the calcium and magnesium to reduce ... around and around in an unhealthful compromising downward spiral.

Stress is so acid-producing that it can acidify an alkaline diet with one surge of adrenaline. Which is one of many very good reasons for the relaxing, system strengthening and integrating, practice of yoga or tai chi.

Cholesterol is a solidified acid, which is warehoused in the body. As much as your organs would like to remove it, they cannot because all the freeways are in gridlock.

Fatty acids make it very challenging for blood to flow, so capillaries clog up and wither away. Because of this, the skin, our largest organ, is not receiving a stimulating flow of nice healthy blood, and loses elasticity becoming wrinkled, just like anything organic left out to dry (think raisins, prunes, dates, figs).

Look at these pictures of blood cells:

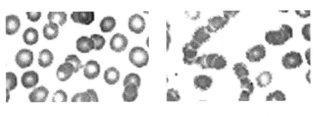

Healthy Blood   Toxic Blood

Blood cells in healthy blood have distance from one another so that they can flow into the smallest of your capillaries, energizing your whole body.

During your deepest sleep, your blood flows everywhere, curing, healing, nurturing, replacing bad with good, calming, stabilizing, doing so much work it's mind boggling to contemplate. No wonder we need to sleep so the blood can work this hard!

Blood cells have a negative—alkaline—charge on the outside and a positive—acid—charge on the inside. Because of this electrical charge, they remain healthy, as the negative charge keeps them at a naturally repelled distance from one another.

A too acidic environment destroys the necessary negative charge in blood and thus the blood becomes coagulated.

Simply stated, over acidity strips your blood of its absolutely necessary negative charge, and if blood is like the second picture, with the cells stuck together, it cannot go everywhere, it does not move wonderfully, it is sticky and sluggish.

One result is poor sleep, and many people wake up depressed, feeling dehydrated, exhausted, and sleepy.

All of your organs are working to keep your blood at its balanced pH, because the whole host will not lonager exist if the blood deviates from its necessary pH.

In short, excess acidity weakens all body systems.

PARASITES

Doctors, researchers, and alternative Health Care professionals agree on one point—disease is caused by imbalance in the body. Imbalance can occur in nutrition, body electricity, body structure, toxicology and/or biology.

Healing chronic illness takes place only when the blood is consistently maintained at a normal, slightly alkaline pH. We live in a world plagued with "microforms"—yeasts, fungii, viruses and molds live within us, eat our glucose, fats and proteins, turns them into poison, then dumps these poisonous excretions within us. If that was not graphic enough, toxic wastes are produced when microforms digest our body.

But microforms cannot survive in an alkaline environment. We need our alkaline minerals to keep an alkaline balance.

Every mineral has its own signature pH level, which allows it to be assimilated by your body. Elements at the lower end of the atomic chart of elements are capable of being assimilated over a broader pH range. Elements higher on the chart can only be assimilated in a narrower pH range.

If your pH is unbalanced, your body will reject most minerals.

Iodine, for instance, is high up on the atomic scale and requires near perfect pH in order to be assimilated into the body. Iodine is necessary for a healthy thyroid gland. Arthritis, heart attacks, diabetes, cancer, depression, obesity, and fatigue have all been connected to thyroid problems. If the pH is unbalanced, then iodine (among others) cannot be absorbed.

> *Those willing to look again, and with clear eyes, will be rewarded with the secrets to permanent health. We can heal ourselves by changing the environment inside our bodies. Potentially harmful invaders, then, will have nowhere to grow and will become harmless."*
>
> **Dr. Robert O. Young, The pH Miracle**

MINERALS

Alkaline minerals include calcium, potassium, magnesium, and sodium. Acid minerals include chlorine, sulfur, and phosphorus, which form hydrochloric acid, sulfuric acid, and phosphoric acid.

Calcium can replace lost alkalinity that had been raided in the acidic body, but the problem is that calcium is very difficult to absorb if your body is excessively acid. Where it is most needed is where it will most likely not be absorbed in supplement form.

An unbalanced acidic system will always search for calcium but unless the cause is corrected, the search continues in vain.

While it is commonly understood that the body needs calcium to build bones, what perhaps is not as commonly known is that bones are a complex matrix of many different minerals. If all the required minerals are not present, strong bones cannot be built. There are at least 18 key bone-building nutrients essential for optimum bone health. It is easier to destroy bone through excess acidity than it is to rebuild bone.

If body fluids are acid they will seek alkaline minerals to react with—such as sodium, potassium, zinc, iron, calcium. These will be robbed from the liver, muscles, ligaments and bones, etc., if too little is available in the diet.

The body's internal fluids—interstitial, cerebro-spinal, and lymphatic fluid, liver bile, etc.—are all slightly alkaline. The only exception is hydrochloric acid produced by the stomach, for the initial task of breaking down what comes into it.

When food is consumed and metabolized, all of it is not used up. A residue, referred to as "ash" remains. Digestion oxidizes foods in much the same way as if they were burned except that it involves enzymes operating at low temperatures.

As mentioned previously, although a lemon tastes acid, and is acid, its ash is alkaline. Lemon breaks down into carbohydrates that further break down into carbon dioxide and water, leaving an alkaline ash consisting of sodium, potassium, calcium, and other mineral salts.

Cells naturally produce acid as a by-product. This acid waste matter is reduced to carbon dioxide and water, and removed from the body. Proteins also leave an acid ash (consisting of phosphates, sulphates and nitrates).

The net effect of eating animal or vegetable protein is to increase acidity, and the body must eliminate this acid waste, but this type of acid ash cannot be eliminated through the lungs as carbon dioxide and water in the same way as with cellular metabolism.

The body must buffer the ash with alkaline substances to neutralize it. Buffering takes place both inside and outside of the cell, while most of the buffering occurs in the blood itself. Supplementing the diet with appropriate alkalizing agents has been shown in clinical studies to be highly beneficial in elevating pH by replenishing alkaline mineral and enzyme reserves.

> *"pH paper strips to measure acid/alkaline pH balance belong in every family medicine kit, right beside the thermometer and bandages."*
> **Dr. R. Dunne**

WHAT CAN I DO?

• Take a calcium supplement in an ionic form for fast, efficient assimilation.

• To see how acidic you are, do urine and saliva pH testing

• A simple test to see if you're too acidic is to pinch the skin on your back. If you are acidic, you'll discover that you almost cannot get a purchase on the skin on your back which is because of being too acidic and, again, the body is doing everything in its power to move the acid away from internal organs and out to the fat layer under the skin, filling the fat cells with the poisonous acid.

Chapter Five

A Bit Of Biology

"Now we depart from health in just the proportion to which we have allowed our alkalis to be dissipated by introduction of acid- forming food in too great amount ... It may seem strange to say that all disease is the same thing, no matter what its myriad modes of expression, but it is verily so."
Dr. William Howard Hay,
A New Health Era, 1933

An overly acid environment in your body is also called "acidosis." Acidosis

Dr. Keith Scott-Mumby *provides the following metaphor, which I*

is believed to be the foundation of all disease. Understanding the simple process of alkalizing your body and the important role a properly alkalized body plays in restoring and maintaining your overall health is critically important. Our organs and glands function in exact proportion to the amount of alkalinity in our system.

ACIDOSIS CAN CAUSE:

Cardiovascular damage / Weight gain, obesity and diabetes / Bladder conditions / Kidney stones / Immune deficiency/Acceleration of free radical damage / Hormonal problems / Premature aging/ Osteoporosis and joint pain/Aching muscles and lactic acid buildup/Low energy and chronic fatigue ...

Slow digestion and elimination/Yeast/fungal overgrowth/Lack of energy and fatigue / Lower body temperature / Tendency to get infections / loss of drive, joy / enthusiasm/Depressive tendencies/Easily stressed/Pale complexion/Headaches/Inflammation of the corneas and eyelids. /Loose and painful teeth/Inflamed, sensitive gums ...

Mouth and stomach ulcers / Cracks at the corners of the lips / Excess stomach acid / Gastritis / Nails are thin and split easily / Hair looks dull, has split ends, and falls out / Dry skin / Skin easily irritated / Leg cramps and spasms / Acne / Dizziness / Joint pains that travel / Food allergies / Chemical sensitivities or odors, gas, heat ...

Hyperactivity / Panic attacks / Premenstrual and menstrual cramping / PMS / Bloating / Heartburn / Diarrhea / Constipation / Hot urine / Panting / Rapid heartbeat / Irregular heartbeat / White coated tongue / Hard to wake up / Excess Head mucus / Metallic taste in mouth / Cold sores ...

find wonderfully apt and graphically clarifying:

"Pretend your have a goldfish in a bowl, and one day you saw the goldfish was looking very unhealthy. You also notice that the water the fish is swimming in is dirty. What makes more sense? To take the fish out of its water and try to heal it? Or to change its water? When you change the water, the fish will get healthy."

The fact that the goldfish is unhealthy is a symptom of the unhealthy environment. Treating the fish and putting it back in an unhealthy medium will not make the fish healthy.

Depression / Loss of memory / Loss of concentration / Migraine headaches/ insomnia / Disturbance in smell, vision, taste / Asthma / Bronchitis / Hay Fever / Ear Aches / Hives / Swelling / Viral infections (cold, flu) / Bacterial Infections (staph, strep) / Fungal infections (candida albicans, athlete's foot, vaginal) ...

Impotence / Urethritis/Cystitis/Urinary infection/Colitis / Hair loss / Psoriasis / Endemetriosis / Stuttering/Numbness and tingling / Sinusitis / Crohn's disease ...

Schizophrenia / Learning Disabilities / Hodgkin's Disease / Systemic Lupus / Erythematosis / MS / Sarcoidosis / Rheumatoid arthritis / Myasthenia Gravis / Scieroderma / Leukemia / Tuberculosis / Other forms of cancer.

These are all symptoms of the lovely garden of you being overly acidic, or suffering from acidosis—and, whenever your see the terms acidic, acid-forming or over acid, please remember that means "toxic."

Here are some possible influences of acidosis on your organs:

The heart is one of the most alkaline-dependent organs in the body. Heartbeat is altered by acid wastes, which also robs the blood of proper oxygenation followed by the degeneration of the heart. An alkaline system creates an ideal heart environment.

Digestive difficulties (belching, bloating, sensitivity at the waist, intestinal gas, regurgitation, hiccups, lack or limitation of appetite, nausea, vomiting, diarrhea, constipation, colic in children) may indicate vagus nerve problems and possible hiatal hernia, which can produce acid residue throughout the system. Hiatal hernia quickly reduces necessary hydrochloric acid in the stomach. Without proper hydrochloric acid breakdown of foods, the foods become too acidic, which causes the hiatal hernia to react, which reduces hydrochloric, etc., etc., *ad nauseam* ... literally!

It is very interesting how much modern day medicine is intent upon pulling the fish from the bowl (treating symptoms) rather than changing the water (addressing the cause of the symptom).

The liver has over three hundred functions, including processing acid toxins from the blood and producing numerous alkaline enzymes for the system. It is also your first line of defense against poisons. All the nourishment obtained through the gastrointestinal tract enters the blood via the liver. The load on the liver can become overwhelming when acid waste products are constantly floating in the blood. If the liver becomes too congested with protein acid wastes, unfortunately, death ensues.

The pancreas depends on your alkaline diet, as it's functions reduce excess acidity and regulate blood sugar. To have proper blood sugar, you must maintain an alkaline-forming diet.

The Peyer's Patches, in the upper portion of the small intestines are crucial to life. They are essential for proper assimilation of food and producing lymphocytes for the lymphatic system's wide-ranging nodal network. They also produce large amounts of the enzyme "chyle," which is a major alkalizing substance. The uninterrupted flow of chyle into the system is crucial. Too much acid waste production from acid-forming foods is a great burden on the Peyer's Patches, which lessens the production of chyle.

"My discovery of the truth ... that acidosis is the cause of all so-called diseases ... step by step, line upon line, precept upon precept, here a little and there a little ... I learned through years of research that localized or systemic acidosis is the true general cause of all disease and must be autogenerated. And if disease is due to autogenerated acids, what is the cause of that autogeneration? I realized that there must be a physical or emotional disturbance to organized matter before it can begin its disorganization. And when matter begins to disorganize, it gives rise to autogenerated acids. This is true for All matter!"

Dr. Robert O. Young,
Sick and Tired, Reclaim Your Inner Terrain

In an adult, about one liter of blood per minute passes through the kidneys. The kidneys' job is to keep the blood alkaline and extract acid.

Kidneys that are over-stressed with too much acidity will often create kidney stones, composed of waste acid cells and mineral salts, all clumped together in a waste acid substance. Reducing acid-forming agents and life style improves your chances of avoiding this painful condition.

The colon must be kept clean of accumulated acid wastes. Poisons collect on the colon walls and in both cases of diarrhea or constipation will harden and reabsorb into the bloodstream.

There are 600-700 lymph glands in your body. Lymph fluid, which flows best in an alkaline environment, carries nutrition to the cells and removes acid waste products.

When the body is overly acidic, lymph slows, creating chronic, long-term, life-threatening situations. In an acidic environment, the lymph dries and begins to form from small to large adhesions throughout the tissues, which interfere with lymph fluid flow and blood flow, increasing tissue acid storage.

Not drinking enough water will also slow the lymph, and waste products from foods not properly digested are reabsorbed into general circulation via the lymphatic ducts of the small intestine, bowel movements that do not completely clear the body of its daily poisons are also reabsorbed.

It has been suggested by numerous cutting edge health care professionals that even cancer is not a disease, but symptomology of disorder, that the affect of metabolic acids and the catarrh that has built up in the blood and then dumped into the tissues significantly damages the white blood cells' ability to remove the acids (along with the cells the acids destroy) out of the body through healthy elimination means.

When toxins accumulate beyond the toleration point, a crisis takes place and the poison or acid is eliminated through the skin, i.e., the third kidney, systemic latent tissue acidosis. What we call disease is the symptoms produced by the body eliminating acids through the mucous membrane.

When this elimination is through the mucous membrane of the nose, you say you have a cold. When this happens year in and year out, the mucous membrane eventually thickens and ulcerates and bones enlarge and close the passages, and hay fever or asthma may develop.

When the throat or tonsils or the respiratory passages become the focus of acidity, we have croup, tonsillitis, pharyngitis, laryngitis, bronchitis, asthma, pneumonia, etc.

Dementia, Parkinson's, Alzheimer's, muddled

thinking, forgetfulness, depression result when the acids locate in the cranial cavity.

> *"The proper way to study disease is to study health and every influence favorable ... to its continuance. Disease is but perverted health. (Therefore) disease cannot be its own cause, neither can it be its own cure and certainly not is own prevention!*

> *"After twenty-five years of research I have discovered that the human organism is alkaline by design but acidic by function. Eliminate the metabolic acids from our tissues and organs and we can live a long and healthy life free from all sickness and disease! The one treatment is to alkalize our body."*
> **Dr. Robert O. Young**

WHAT CAN I DO?

- As quantum physicists are discovering, looking with intention manifests that intention—be mindful!
- Dissolve in your hot bath 2 or 3 cups Epsom salts and 1/4 cup of baking soda, soak for 20-30 minutes. Or use sea salt. Or a cup of baking soda ... all are soothing and alkalizing.
- For jet lag, drink down a couple glasses of water and then continue to hydrate—a lot!—with more glasses of water. Dr. Baroody's formula: 1 teaspoon chlorophyll power in 8 ounces water for every 2 hours of travel, reduces both jet lag and fear of flying.
- Deep diaphragmatic breathing, yoga, tai chi and detoxification processes dredge out acid wastes. Take steam baths and saunas to dredge skin, your largest eliminatory organ.
- Do a body scrub daily before showering or bathing with Dead Sea salt scrubs and mud wrap massage.
- Use herbal oils in the steam room and negative ion generators.
- Kidney and bladder cleanse with herbal teas, and alkaline water to eliminate wastes and toxins.
- Meditation

- Yoga, and/or tai chi to center, calm, heal, oxygenate, and to fully engage your life force
- Moderate exercise is alkalizing to the body. Excessive exercise (past the point of exhaustion) can create a lactic acid buildup.
- Important for cancer treatment/prevention are the alkaline trace minerals rubidium and cesium.

> *"Exercising with good aerobic activity to just before the point of exhaustion creates an alkaline response because of increased oxygenation. If we exercise past that point, the body releases excess acidity."*
> **Dr. Theodore Baroody, Alkalize or Die**

Chapter Six

Emotions & pH Balance

"I choose to be happy."
Dr. Wayne Dyer

Have you ever been so upset with someone or something that you felt sick?

All negative emotions create an acidic environment. Sayings such as, "don't let that eat at you" are based in a deep, true,

Dr. Baroody has an *exercise which he calls "Hold One Point" which is both relaxing and empowering.*

Visualize a circle about the size of a quarter in your stomach, an inch below

perhaps somewhat unconscious understanding of the power of emotions—and how they can affect your essential health.

It has been suggested that fear is the underlying cause of most disease. Fear manifests anger. Anger becomes hate. Hate can be all-consuming if you permit it to be the boss of you, instead of you being the boss of you, and your emotions.

As you suffer you will generate an acidic pH in your body, until it takes up what it is being taught, and begins to fall apart in an acidic melt down.

Love, peace, joy, calmness, forgiveness, something to believe in, a passion for life, and something within your life that is yours and yours alone to feel passionate about are ways to re-alkalize yourself.

STRESS

When your system is placed in a fighting posture even though no adversary is directly present—such as a traffic jam, the evening news, etc., excessive hormones are generated, without the outlet anticipated by the body.

Your muscles contract, and your digestive circuits are rerouted. Even alkaline-forming foods become acidic under these circumstances, so the cell does not get its oxygen, and breaks down. Blood and lymph flows are redirected to the "crisis." All of this acid action becomes something that we ultimately feel. We name it stress.

"The secret of establishing and maintaining an alkaline-forming state of being is in the form of service. This does not mean that you must give everything you have away. It is the essential way you treat your neighbor and yourself."
Dr. Theodore Baroody,
Alkalize or Die

your navel. Imagine the dot decreasing in size by one-half, then by one-half again, and then by one-half again without letting it disappear. This focus centers the mind and quiets the body. You will sense the quiet hook up of your mind and your bodily center, and probably discover that what was distressing, bothering, angering, or worrying you simply is not nearly as looming as it was.

TRAUMA

Physical trauma produces a very real acid response in your body. To be in a car accident—even if you walk away from it—with muscular, ligament and tissue trauma, will probably cause an acidic reaction of around two.

All during the time it takes to heal, there is acid-forming reaction, and so one needs to be particularly attentive to providing alkaline-forming food, water, relaxation and activities.

There are also the acidic producing psychological aspects of trauma—time off work, which might cause anxiety, worry, insomnia, etc., stress from doctor's visits, and the very acidic energy and stress surrounding dealing with insurance and attorneys.

Counter each negative, acidic event with a surrounding shield of calm, peace, and release, supported by alkaline diet and beverage, and much rest.

Remind yourself that stress, worry and anxiety will not change the outcome, and the very strongest position you have is to support alkaline balance and be healthy!

Surgery is also traumatic, so if you have a surgery pending, be sure to include some alkalizing items in your overnight bag—enriching, or amusing books you've been meaning to read, music that soothes and relaxes, etc., and then make, to the degree that you're empowered under the circumstances, alkaline dietary choices.

Perhaps you have heard of the Social Readjustment Scale, with 43 measurements of life stressors. On this self-evaluations test, you give yourself points for various life experiences that cause stress, examples being: the death of a spouse at 100 points, mortgage at 35 points, Christmas at 12 points, and add the points up, with scoring as follows, to indicate the likelihood of physical and mental health issues:

Low < 149
Mild = 150-200
Moderate = 200-299
Major >300

(This copyrighted instrument can be found readily on the internet under either the title, as above, or the authors, Dr. T. H. Holmes and Dr. R. H. Rahe.)

The objective of taking into consideration the information you may glean from taking this test is not to add to your stress, but to realize that if you have a high score, it is important to support a calming, alkaline-forming diet and environment.

Another tension relaxer, calming alkalizing action, borrowed from reflexology, is to massage your feet in their solar plexus relieving location, as shown on this graphic:

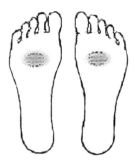

"Sleep is a sense, and as such is as important
as seeing, tasting, smelling and hearing.
During sleep many acid by-products are
processed and eliminated from the body, in
part through a deeper breathing than we ever
allow ourselves when conscious (an excellent

*reason for yoga and meditation where deep
breathing are part of the discipline). This
deep sleep repair is alkaline producing."*
Dr. Theodore Baroody, Alkalize or Die

WHAT CAN I DO?

• Listen to Music—but be sure it is music that makes you feel happy, relaxed, enthusiastic, or just, simply good all over. If you are not consciously aware of a general feeling of well-being from the music you're listening to, change the music until you do.

• Silence is also golden.

• Yoga, and/or tai chi, which center, calm, heal, oxygenate, and to fully engage your life force.

• Choose to be happy.

• Alternative healing systems produce alkaline-forming reactions. These include: acupuncture, acupressure, ayurvedic, chiropractic, color and music therapy, talk therapy (counseling), food supplementation, vitamin, minerals, herbology, homeopathy, massage, radionics, reflexology, shiatsu, spiritual healing, yoga, tai chi, and others.

• Also various electrical modalities are alkaline producing, such as diathermy, galvanic, infrared, muscle stimulation, ultrasound, ultraviolet, electrical homeopathy, cold laser acupuncture, magnetic beds, and others.

> *"Our bodies are composed of the same minerals that form the sun and moon. Our hearts are rhythmically tuned to the pulsations of gold and white light that these wonders of God splash so abundantly across the porch of the mind."*
> **Dr. Theodore Baroody, Alkalize or Die**

Chapter Seven

The Anti-Aging Process

*"It is very possible to have continuous
cellular regeneration ... outnumber
cellular degeneration. This equates to
a physical youthening."*
Dr. Theodore Baroody

The accumulation of waste products inside your body is the aging process. So helping your body get rid of the old waste products contributes to keeping you young

*What would happen
to your town if the
garbage collectors went
on strike? Think about
the results after a week
- trash is piling up
around domestic trash
sites, starting to smell.*

and healthy. The reverse aging process has two components:

1. A healthy disposal system

And

2. The function of this disposal system. It pulls the old wastes out from in all the nooks and crannies of your body - joints, fat, etc., where they have been stored, and expels them.

RELEASING ACIDIC WASTES

Aging, in simplest terms, is the body's accumulation of acidic wastes.

In spite of the fact that your cells produce acidic wastes constantly, your body fluids must maintain a slightly alkaline pH.

In order to reduce acidity of the blood, your lungs exhaust carbon dioxide when you breathe, carbonic acid becomes water when carbon dioxide is removed, which is nature's fastest way to reduce blood acidity.

Even with your body's constant labors to dispose of acidic wastes, given the current diet, lifestyle, and environment (over-eating, over-drinking, overwork, over-indulgence, inadequate sleep, inadequate exercise, inadequate water consumption, smoking, pollution, low alkaline diet, stress, anxiety, worry, etc., etc., and etc., all of which are acid-forming) we still produce more acidic wastes than our bodies can get rid of.

What the body then does with this excess acid is to convert the liquid acids into solid acids. It gets quite busy making cholesterol, fatty acids, kidney stones, phosphates, uric acid, urates, and other damaging solid acids. The number one contributor to aging is that your body is not (and cannot if continually bombarded with more excess acids) disposing of all these internally generated wastes and toxins, accumulating in your body.

After two weeks people try to dispose of their own garbage by moving it about, but everyone is moving their garbage around so the situation does not improve. The garbage pile-up continues to mount, looking ever more horrible, and creating a terrible stench.

It also poses a serious health concern due to unsanitary conditions. Gradually, no one can drive around as the streets are piled with garbage. What does this picture look like after a year?

Now imagine the city of your organs and arteries and bones and muscles, in short, your interior, experiencing

The reason your body works so hard to make solid acids of these toxins is its valiant efforts to keep them from doing the harm they do when in liquid form—just in the same way you reach for the paper towels when there's a spill.

Also mixed with these organic acids are inorganic acid minerals, such as chlorine, phosphor, and sulfur, which are part of acidic foods—meats, grains and root crops.

ARE THERE SOLUTIONS?

Yes! Here are actions you can begin today!

1. *Reduce acidic foods considerably.* Refer to the Alkaline-Acidic chart in the back of the book to become familiar with the wisest, healthiest alkaline food choices.

2. *Increase alkaline, anti-aging foods.* Namely, fruits and vegetables, which contain those wonderful and much needed inorganic alkaline minerals. The primary inorganic minerals are: calcium, magnesium, sodium, and potassium. Become familiar with your favorite foods that supply these minerals. Or develop new favorites!

3. *Drink acid free, alkaline water.*

These changes of habit will gradually elevate your blood pH and the aging processes (and the diseases connected with them) can slow, and even reverse, naturally.

WHAT CAN I DO?

• Harmonize your diet and emotions with your quiet, centered self to stimulate cellular regeneration.

• Yoga, and/or tai chi to center, calm, heal, oxygenate, and to fully engage your life force.

• Meditate.

• Everything else that is suggested in this book.

year in and year out acid garbage pile up.

It is long past time to re-negotiate the contract with the garbage collectors and pay them their much deserved alkaline "wages." Get your exquisite city shining and healthy and all the arterial road ways open and clean again!

"It is what stays in our bodies as waste that creates our over-acidic condition and causes us to age prematurely."

Sang Whang, Reverse Aging

Chapter Eight

Healing Crisis

"Cultivate your own garden."
Voltaire

Remarkable things begin to happen to the body as well as the mind when a person decides to make an improvement in the quality of food consumed. The amazing, healing, intelligence present in every cell begins to manifest almost immediately. When the quality of food coming into the body is of higher quality than the tissue that the body is made of, the body begins to discard the lower grade materials to integrate the superior materials now provided, to make new and healthier tissue.

When the use of toxic foods and beverages is suddenly stopped, a "healing crisis" occurs, headaches, stiffness, pains in new places, rashes, and fatigue are all possible.

The healing crisis is due to the healthier, slower action of the heart, the resting phase that follows the stimulation of more rapid heart action forced on the body by stimulants.

During a healing crisis, the body is discarding toxins, which are removed from the tissues and transported through the blood stream. Before the toxic agents reach their final destination for elimination, they register as pain.

Examples of lower quality foods are foods that have undergone more preparation. Some spices and salt tend to be more stimulating than less prepared and more natural foods. Animal protein from mammals, fowl, fish etc., is more stimulating than cheeses, nuts and vegetable proteins.

Usually, within three days the painful symptoms begin to abate, and you will likely feel stronger than you have in a long time. This initial healing crisis lasts from ten days to perhaps several weeks, depending, in part, on the level of contamination, and the clarity of resolve of the individual to stick with the cure, followed by an increase of strength, diminishing stress, and a profound sense of well-being.

During the initial phase of healing, the energy that is usually in the external parts of the body such as the muscles and skin, move to the vital internal organs and start reconstruction.

This shunting of power to the internal region produces fatigue in the muscles, which you may be inclined to interpret, understandably, as weakness. However, your power is actually increasing, being used for rebuilding the more critical organs, so less of it is available for muscular work.

During this time of regeneration, get a lot of rest. Sleep as much as your body is asking to be allowed to sleep, and let the healing continue in a constructively peaceful environment. This is a crucial phase, and resorting to stimulants and stimulation will defeat the regeneration.

As you continue on the improved diet and gradually raise your food quality, your body begins a process called "retracing." Your cells say, "Look at the wonderful materials coming in! Let's get rid of this garbage and build strong new organs."

So it gets excess bile out of the liver and gall bladder and sends it to the intestines for elimination. It moves sludge out of the arteries, veins, and capillaries. It cleans up arthritic deposits on the joints. It cleans out preservatives such as aspirin, sleeping pills and drugs, along with masses of fat.

During the first phase of the healing crisis, called catabolism, the accent is on elimination and breaking down defective tissue. Wastes are discarded rapidly and new tissue is made from the new food, and you will experience weight loss.

This phase is followed by a second stage of stabilization, and your weight probably levels off. During this phase, the amount of waste material being discarded daily is equal to the amount of tissue being formed which occurs after the excess of obstructing material in the tissues has been removed.

After this stage follows a third phase, anabolism, which is a building up period. By this time, most of the toxic wastes have been discarded.

If you have had tendencies in the past to skin rashes or eruptions, you will likely eliminate poisons and harmful drugs through the skin with new rashes and eruptions. If you go to a doctor who is not familiar with this aspect of nutrition and healing, the doctor is likely diagnose it as an allergy.

Remember, your body is "retracing." The skin is becoming more alive, throwing out poisons rapidly. Headaches may occur, fever and/or colds may manifest, the skin may break out, there may be a short interval of bowel discomfort, feeling tired and weak, a disinclination to exercise, nervousness, irritability, depression, frequent urination, etc.

But if you know that these symptoms mean that your healing efforts are working, you will hopefully feel encouraged and "brave," and see it through to your happy, healthy destination! The symptoms are part of healing, so don't try to cure a cure.

These symptoms are likely to vary according to the material being discarded, the condition of the organs involved in the elimination, and the amount of energy you have available. The more you rest and sleep, the milder the symptoms will be and the more quickly resolved.

Your body is becoming younger and healthier every day. You are providing a one-way ticket for wastes that, if retained, would have brought pain and disease.

Your body is cyclical in nature, and your health will return in gradually diminishing cycles. For example, you may start a better diet and for a while you feel much better. After some time, a symptom occurs—you may feel nauseous for a day, then after a day, you feel better than ever before, and all goes fine for a while. Then you suddenly develop a cold, feel chills, and lose your appetite. After about two or three days you suddenly develop an itch or rash. You do not take anything special for it. This rash flares up, gets worse, and continues for ten days, and immediately subsides.

Reactions become milder as the body becomes purer, with longer and longer periods of feeling better than ever before, until you reach a plateau of vibrant, happy health, with a body reveling in not having to constantly battle to maintain its own best pH balance!

WHAT CAN I DO?
- Drink lots and lots of water.
- Implement dietary changes gradually.
- Keep in touch with your Health Care provider.
- Congratulate yourself heartily and frequently for your focus on self-improvement!

Chapter Nine

Old MacDonald Had a Farm

"That which is built on alkalinity sustains,
that which is built on acidity falls away.
Mother Earth calls out for the
alkaline way of life."
Dr. Theodore Baroody, Alkalize or Die

Inadequate mineral supply to our bodies is extremely common because of the depletion of minerals in our agricultural land. The supply and absorption of adequate miner-

Animals
Half of all antibiotics and steroids produced are fed to domestic animals. Herbicides and pesticides are sprayed on their food. This acid-forming,

als to your body determines your health as it determines the conductivity of electricity. Electrical conductivity is the basis of an effective nervous system, which, in turn, monitors and reports on how well your various organs and subsystems are doing, which are also, essentially, electrical entities.

The simple solution to this problem on every level is to eat vegetables and fruits, the more of them fresh the better.

FARMING

Every living thing is an electrical system—a balance of positive and negative charge that keeps that system healthy and alive. Our diet is overwhelmingly acid-forming, which is a positive charge. We're burning up! We need more negative, alkalizing charge (i.e. negative ions) to run smoothly.

There is a direct correlation between higher alkaline-forming and higher natural sugars ("appropriate body fuel") in fruits, vegetables, and grains. Healthy fruits and veggies taste "sweeter" in the most attractive, and pleasant manner.

When food crops are at optimum alkalinity with natural sugars there are virtually no disease or insect infestations. The body of food crops is just like your body. When it is alkaline, disease and opportune creatures cannot infiltrate. Dr. Anderson, author of *The Anatomy of Life and Energy in Agriculture* writes that what is put in our soils is nitrogen and potash, which are acid-forming, and what is needed is calcium and phosphate, alkaline-forming.

The vicious circle is that the farmer sprays to kill insects, the spray makes the crop more acidic and the insects work arduously to eradicate the acidic foods, as is their function according to the Law of Nature. The objective of Nature is that more complicated animals— that would include humans – be left with only the best produce.

poison remains in their bodies.

Arsenic is fed to chickens to avoid quick spreading virus. Ninety percent of commercially raised chickens show evidence of cancer. Beaks are cut off the bird and they are force fed with tubes, then they are electrocuted. If the stress of, say, being late for work will cause you to have an acid rush, imagine what this compilation of abuse and torture to these creatures manifests in their bodies as acid residue.

Turkey breasts are bleached to look whiter—an acid-forming process, and meat is dyed red with acid-forming nitrate to look more red, which breaks down to nitrosamines, which are cancer causing agents.

The insects multiply their populations in an effort to answer to the demand of ever-expanding volumes of acidic crops and produce that is only fit for insect consumption and the farmers go out and spray to kill insects, which makes the crop more acidic and the insects work arduously to eradicate the acidic foods, as is their function, according to the Law of Nature ... around and around again.

Agricultural chemicals are all acid-forming, therefore, our produce and farm crops no longer contain the necessary minerals and natural sugars we need.

In a study before 1930, farmers lost one-third of their crop to insects. In a study done in the 1980's the farmers lost one-third of their crops to insects—after millions of pounds of acidic, soil-depleting pesticides were poured on crops. In that fifty years all we had accomplished was less nutritious, acid-forming crops, while adding profound amounts of pollution to the planet, and skyrocketing food prices to pay for it all.

USE OF ALKALINE WATER ON DAIRY FARMS

With the advent of electrolysis water treatment in the Japanese marketplace, electrolysis alkaline water was introduced into dairy farms, which is finally beginning to make an impression on American dairy farms, and in other countries as well.

Japan, having learned the positive health benefits that were acquired through human consumption of alkaline water, used it in place of tap water as the sole source of water for dairy cows in a large scale experimentation, and some of the results, obtained from 27 dairy farms and a group of veterinarians follow:

- An increase in milk output by 18% - 28%
- A notable improvement in the quality of milk
- Minimized injury to the udder
- Decrease in diarrhea cases
- Strengthening of the legs
- Increased appetite including even in older cows
- Well digested foods
- Beautiful sheen on cow hides
- Less mineral supplements needed to be added to the feed
- Extended productive life span of the cows
- Improved fertility rate and reduced still births
- Newborn calves exposed to alkali water matured faster
- Improved liver condition
- Tremendously improved health, very little

sickness
- Elimination of strong waste odors
- Fewer visits by veterinarians
- **No** adverse conditions noted with use of alkali water

WHAT CAN I DO?

- Buy produce from your weekend farmers market, which tends to be populated by what I've christened, "produce artists." They are generally passionate about what they grow.
- They grow organic, they put their own intention, energy and focus into their crop, and every single "produce artist" I've ever talked with (being an avid farmer's market attendee) has either voluntarily mentioned praying over or for the produce, or answered (perhaps somewhat shyly) in the affirmative when I've asked if they pray for their crop.
- *Do not* support factory farming. And, even better ....
- Maintain a plant-based diet.
- Insist on organic everything.
- Why not grow your own?

About the Author

It's about You—but here's a few words about me to inspire your trust in what I write ....

I know that a happy, kind, productive world evolves from happy, kind, productive, individual people.

The goal of my writing is to help clear your path to joyful productivity, in the glow of a healthy, contented, and meaningful life.

A Bit of Bio ....
I received my Doctorate from the University of California at Irvine in the School of Social Sciences, with a focus on psychology and ethnography. I've always been relentlessly curious about how people think, and how those thoughts make them feel.

After I submitted my doctoral dissertation, I moved to the Pacific Northwest, to write and to have a small private psychotherapy practice in a tiny town not much bigger than a village.

I worked with many amazing people, and witnessed astounding emotional, psychological, and spiritual, healing. It was a wonderful experience. But after twenty plus years, I realized it was time to put my focus on my writing, wherein I could potentially help greater numbers of people. Where I could meet *you!*

I live on ten acres of forest with a few domestic and numerous wild creatures. Along with creating an ever-growing inventory of books, my writing has appeared in hundreds of online and print publications.

Your support of my writing helps support ten acres of natural forest, and all its resident fauna. All the creatures and I thank you!

Questions, comments, observations, reviews? *I'd love to hear from you!*:

Blythe@BlytheAyne.com

www.BlytheAyne.com

NOTE:
You will find an Alkaline-Acid Chart on the following pages. I've arranged the chart with alkaline food and beverage items first. Although you're likely to see this chart elsewhere in the reverse order, because the pH Scale goes from 1 to 14, with 1 being the most acidic, I've placed alkaline items first, as our goal is to focus on a more alkaline diet, and I've made the *good things to eat* show first on the chart.

ANOTHER NOTE:
This content is not intended to be medical advice or instructions for medical diagnosis or treatment. Nothing in these contents should be considered to diagnose, treat, cure, or prevent disease without the supervision of a qualified healthcare provider.

———————

CATEGORY	Alkaline		Acid	Chart	Acid	High Acid
	High Alkaline	Alkaline	Low Alkaline	Low Acid	Acid	High Acid
BEANS VEGETABLES LEGUMES	Asparagus, Broccoli, Onions, Vegetable Juices, Raw Spinach, Garlic, Barley Grass, Bamboo Shoots, Beets, Cilantro, Ginger, Parsley	Okra, Squash, Green Beans, Celery, Lettuce, Zucchini, Sweet Potato, Carob, Chard, Cucumber	Carrots, Corn, Cabbage, Mushroom, Peas, Cauliflower, Turnip, Potato Skin, Olives, Soybeans, Tomatoes, Tofu, Brussels sprouts	Cooked Spinach, Kidney, Black, Red, White, Beans	Potatoes (without skins), Pinto Beans, Navy Beans, Lima Beans	
FRUIT	Lemons, Watermelon, Limes, Grapefruit, Mangoes, Papayas	Dates, Figs, Melons, Grapes, Papaya, Kiwi, Berries, Apples, Pears, Raisins	Oranges, Bananas, Cherries, Pineapple, Peaches, Avocados	Plums, Processed Fruit Juices	Sour Cherries, Rhubarb, Canned Fruit	Blueberries, Cranberries, Prunes, Sweetened Fruit Juice
GRAINS CEREALS			Amaranth, Millet, Lentils, Sweet corn, Wild Rice, Quinoa	Rye Bread, Sprouted Wheat Bread, Spelt, Brown Rice	White Rice, Corn, Buckwheat, Oats, Rye	Wheat, White Bread, Pastries, Biscuits, Pasta
MEAT					Liver, cold water fish	Beef, Pork, Turkey, Chicken, Lamb, Goat, Deer, Shellfish

EGGS DAIRY		Breast Milk	Soy Cheese, Soy Milk, Goat Milk, Goat Cheese, Whey	Eggs, Butter, Yogurt, Buttermilk, Cottage Cheese, Cream	Raw Milk	Cheese, Homogenized Milk, Ice Cream, Custard
NUTS SEEDS	Almonds		Chestnuts, Coconut, Brazil nuts, Hazelnuts	Pumpkin, Sesame, Sunflower Seeds	Pecans, Cashews, Pistachios	Peanuts, Walnuts
OILS	Olive Oil	Flax Seed Oil, Coconut Oil	Canola Oil	Corn Oil, Sunflower Oil, Margarine, Lard		
BEVERAGES	Herb Teas, Lemon Water	Green Tea	Ginger Tea	Tea, Cocoa	Coffee, Wine	Beer, Liquor, Soft Drinks
SWEETENERS CONDIMENTS	Stevia	Maple Syrup, Rice Syrup	Raw Honey, Raw Sugar	Processed Honey	White Sugar, Brown Sugar, Molasses, Jam, Ketchup, Mayonnaise, Mustard, Vinegar	Artificial Sweeteners, Chocolate
OTHER	magnetized water, ionized water, pH balanced water, green juices, most spices, Herbs, Bee Pollen, Umebosi				White Pasta	All Drugs, Medicinal and Street, Pesticides, Herbicides, Distilled Water

DICTIONARY:

Anabolism – the energy-requiring, constructive process, by which living cells convert simple substances into more complex compounds, especially living matter.

Catabolism – The breakdown of organic nutrients in a cell in energy-yielding reactions.

Chlorella – collective name for a single celled algae. It has chlorophyll in its cell and looks green when gathered. It is bacteriostatic, that is, it is capable of inhibiting reproduction of bacteria.

CFCs – Chlorofluorocarbons – A hydrocarbon in which some or all of the hydrogen atoms have been replaced by chlorine and fluorine. Fluorocarbons are used as a feedstock, as a refrigerant, as a solvent and as a blowing agent of plastic foam. Believed to be responsible for depleting the Earth's diminishing ozone layer.

Hado – A Japanese word meaning "wavelength." The vibrational pattern at the atomic level in all matter, employed in the research and healing work of Dr. Masuru Emoto and others.

Homeopath – A physician who treats disease using minute doses of natural substances that would, in a healthy person, elicit the symptoms of the disease being treated.

Hydroxyl ion – Negatively charged species of chemical formula, OH - . Neutral water (pH 7) contains 10-7 mol L-1 hydroxyl ions. Dissolution of bases in water leads to an increase in the hydroxyl ion concentration, and thus an increase in the pH.

Interfacial Tissues – relating to or situated at an interface; tissue between two layers.

Motilin – A 22-amino-acid peptide produced in the mucosa of the small intestine, which stimulates contractions of the stomach and the release of pepsin.

Naturopath – A Naturopathic doctor assists in the health of patients through the application of natural remedies. Naturopaths generally consider their care complementary to the care of a traditional medical professional.

Ptyalin – an amylase secreted in saliva, a digestive enzyme classified as a saccharidase (an enzyme that cleaves polysaccharides), a constituent of pancreatic juice and saliva, needed for the breakdown of long-chain carbohydrates (such as starch) into smaller units.

Toxemia – A condition in which the blood contains toxic substances either of microbial origin or as by-products of abnormal protein metabolism.

Vagus Nerve – The tenth cranial nerve, which originates in the brain stem and affects the heart, lungs, stomach, ears, pharynx, larynx, trachea, esophagus, the majority of the autonomic functions and internal organs.

It is the tenth of twelve paired cranial nerves, and is the only nerve that starts in the brainstem (in the medulla oblongata) and extends down to the abdomen. It is arguably the single most important nerve in the body.

BIBLIOGRAPHY:

Alkalize or Die by Theodore A. Baroody, Holographic Health Press, 1991

Cell Biology of Extracellular Matrix by E.D. Hay, Academic Press, 1981

Health Research by David Marsland, Social Research Today, 1996

Holistic Protocol for the Immune System by Scott J. Gregory, Tree of Life Publications, 2005

Human Energy Systems by Jack Schwarz, E.P. Dutton Publishing, New York, N.Y., 1980

Living in Balance: Reshaping the You Within by Jerry Johnson Ph. D. , 2006

Messages From Water by Dr. Masuru Emoto, Beyond Words Publishing, Inc., 2005

Missing Diagnosis by C. O. Truss, 1985

Molecular Biology of the Cell by Alberts, Et Al., 2002

Mycotoxins in Human and Animal Health by Joseph V. Rodricks, 2004

Prescription for Nutritional Healing by Phyllis Balch, 2006

Social Readjustment Rating Scale, by Drs. T. Holmes and R. Rahe, Pergamon Press, 1971

Staying Healthy with the Seasons by E.M. Haas, Celestial Arts Publishing, Berkeley, California, 1981

The Acid Alkaline Diet for Optimum Health: Restore Your Health by Creating pH Balance in Your Diet, by Christopher Vasey, 2006

The Anatomy of Life & Energy in Agriculture by Anderson, Dr. Arden Kansas City, Missouri Acres, U.S.A., 1989

The Energy Balance Diet: Lose Weight, Control Your Cravings and Even Out Your Energy by Joshua Rosenthal and Tom Monte, 2002

The pH Balance Diet: Restore Your Acid-Alkaline Levels to Eliminate Toxins and Lose Weight, by Bharti Vyas and Suzanne Le Quesne, 2007

The pH Miracle: Balance Your Diet, Reclaim Your Health by Robert O. Young and Shelley Redford Young, 2002

The Possibility of Living 200 Years by F.O. Havens, Health Research, Mokelumne Hill, California, 1896

Toxicology, Biochemistry and Pathology of Mycotoxins by Kenji Uraguchi Kodansha Scientific Books, 1978

Yeast Connection by William G. Crook, 2003

Top 10 foods that fight inflammation Arthritis

1. Broccoli
2. Olive Oil
3. Blueberries
4. Fish
5. Nuts
6. Tart Cherries
7. Kelp
8. Fermented foods
9. Papaya
10. Green tea

5 Worse foods Arthritis + Pain

1. Sugar
2. Nightshade Plants
3. Blackened / Barbeque / charcoal / fried High temp
4. French Fries / Processed Food
5. Bagels / white bread / white pasta
   muffins

Trans facts need to be kept low

CPSIA information can be obtained
at www.ICGtesting.com
Printed in the USA
BVHW03s0227190518
516625BV00006B/49/P

9 780982 783580